Leukaemia And Blood Disease

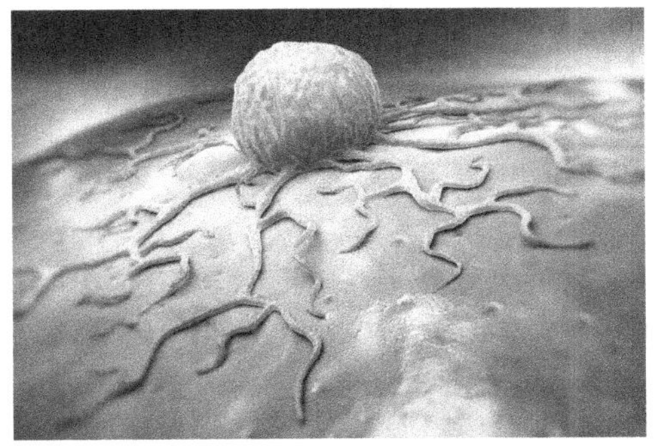

The Comprehensive Guide To Treating and Healing Blood Cancer and Disease

Isaac Hendricks

Copyright © 2023[Isaac Hendricks]

I, [Isaac Hendricks], hereby declare that I am the sole owner and creator of the title "The Road to Recovery: A Guide to Leukaemia and Blood Diseases." I hold all necessary rights and permissions to use this title in connection with my book, which is currently in progress. I certify that this title is original and has not been previously used or registered for any other book or publication. I further affirm that the use of this title does not infringe upon any existing copyright or trademark rights. By signing below, I acknowledge that I am solely responsible for any legal action arising from any claims of infringement or misuse of this title.

Signature:

____

Date:_________________________________

Table of Contents

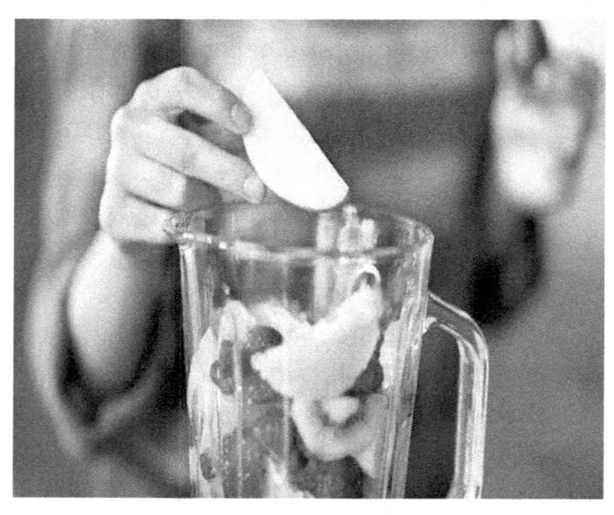

INTRODUCTION

Leukaemia and blood diseases are serious medical conditions that require proper care, treatment, and management. If you or someone you know has been diagnosed with leukaemia or a blood disease, it's essential to understand the condition, its symptoms, and the available treatment options. This guide aims to provide comprehensive information on how to combat and heal from leukaemia and blood diseases.

Leukaemia is a type of cancer that affects the blood-forming cells in the bone marrow. Blood diseases, on the other hand, refer to a range of disorders that affect the production, function, or circulation of blood cells. Some common blood diseases include anaemia, sickle cell disease, thalassemia, and haemophilia.

Leukaemia symptoms vary based on the type and stage of the disease.. Some common symptoms include:

- Fatigue and weakness
- Fever or chills
- Bleeding or bruising easily
- Frequent infections
- Weight loss
- Swollen lymph nodes, spleen, or liver
- Bone pain or tenderness

- Night sweats

If you have any of these symptoms, you should see a doctor right once to get an accurate diagnosis. The diagnosis process may involve a physical exam, blood tests, bone marrow biopsy, and imaging tests. Based on the diagnosis, your healthcare provider will recommend an appropriate treatment plan. Some common treatment options for leukaemia and blood diseases include:

- Chemotherapy: This involves the use of drugs to destroy cancer cells in the body. Chemotherapy can be administered through an IV or taken orally.

- Radiation therapy: This treatment uses high-energy radiation to kill cancer cells. Radiation therapy can be administered both externally and inside.

- Stem cell transplant: This involves replacing damaged stem cells with healthy ones from a donor. Stem cell transplant is typically used for advanced stages of leukaemia.

- Targeted therapy: This involves the use of drugs that specifically target cancer cells based on their genetic makeup. Targeted therapy is often used in combination with chemotherapy or radiation therapy.

- _Immunotherapy:_ This involves using the body's immune system to fight cancer cells. Immunotherapy can be used alone or in combination with other treatments.

In addition to medical treatment, making lifestyle changes can help manage leukaemia and blood diseases. Among the lifestyle adjustments that may be advantageous are:

- _Eating a healthy diet:_ A diet rich in fruits, vegetables, whole grains, and lean protein can help support a healthy immune system and promote overall health. It's essential to avoid foods that may trigger allergies or cause digestive issues. For personalized nutritional advice, consult a qualified nutritionist.

- _Exercising regularly:_ Regular exercise can help improve overall health and reduce stress levels. However, it's essential to consult your healthcare provider before starting any new exercise program to ensure it's safe for your specific condition.

- _Getting enough sleep:_ Aim for 7-8 hours of sleep each night to help support overall health and reduce stress levels. If you have trouble sleeping due to pain or discomfort, consult your healthcare provider for advice on managing these symptoms.

- _Managing stress levels:_ Stress can have a negative impact on overall health and wellbeing.

Consider practising stress-reduction techniques such as meditation, deep breathing exercises, or yoga to help manage stress levels. Consult a mental health professional if you need additional support managing stress related to your condition.

- Quitting smoking: Smoking can increase the risk of developing certain types of cancer and worsen existing conditions such as lung disease or heart disease. Quitting smoking can help improve overall health and reduce the risk of complications related to your condition. Consult your healthcare provider for advice on quitting smoking if you need additional support.

- Avoiding infection: Certain types of leukaemia can make it more difficult for the body to fight off infection. To help prevent infection, avoid close contact with people who are sick, wash your hands frequently with soap and water, and avoid touching your face or mouth without washing your hands first. If you're undergoing chemotherapy or radiation therapy, you may need additional precautions such as avoiding crowds or public places where there is an increased risk of infection. Consult your healthcare provider for personalised advice on preventing infection based on your specific condition and treatment plan.

Overview of Leukaemia and Blood Diseases

Leukaemia and blood diseases are a group of disorders that affect the blood-forming organs, including the bone marrow and lymphatic system. Leukaemia is a type of blood cancer that occurs when the bone marrow produces an excessive number of abnormal white blood cells, which interfere with the production of normal blood cells. Blood diseases, on the other hand, refer to a range of disorders that affect the blood's composition, including anaemia, haemophilia, and sickle cell disease.

In this article, we will provide an overview of leukaemia and blood diseases, including their causes, symptoms, diagnosis, and treatment.

Causes:

The exact causes of leukaemia and blood diseases are not fully understood. However, several factors have been identified as potential risk factors for these disorders. These include exposure to ionising radiation, environmental pollutants, certain viruses (such as HIV), genetic mutations, and chemotherapy or radiation therapy used to treat other cancers or diseases.

Symptoms:

The symptoms of leukaemia and blood diseases can vary depending on the type and stage of the disorder. Common symptoms include fatigue, weakness, fever, weight loss, easy bruising or bleeding, frequent infections, bone pain or tenderness, swollen lymph nodes, and enlargement of the liver or spleen.

Diagnosis:

The diagnosis of leukaemia and blood diseases involves a series of tests and examinations to confirm the presence and type of disorder. These may include a complete blood count (CBC), bone marrow aspiration and biopsy, cytogenetic analysis (karyotyping), fluorescence in situ hybridization (FISH), molecular genetic testing (PCR), and imaging studies such as CT scans or MRI.

Treatment:

The treatment for leukaemia and blood diseases depends on several factors, including the type and stage of the disorder, age and overall health of the patient, and preferences for treatment. Common treatments include chemotherapy (the use of drugs to destroy cancer cells), radiation therapy (the use of high-energy radiation to destroy cancer cells), stem cell transplantation (the replacement of damaged bone marrow with healthy stem cells), targeted therapy (the use of drugs that specifically target cancer cells), immunotherapy (the use of drugs that stimulate the patient's immune system to fight cancer cells), and supportive care (the use of medications to manage symptoms such as pain or infection).

Leukaemia and blood diseases are complex disorders that require careful diagnosis and individualised treatment plans. While significant progress has been made in understanding these disorders and developing effective treatments, further research is needed to improve outcomes for patients with these conditions. By continuing to study these disorders at the molecular level and develop new therapies based on our understanding of their underlying mechanisms, we can hope to make significant strides in improving outcomes for patients with leukaemia and blood diseases in the future.

Importance of Lifestyle in Healing

Leukaemia and other blood diseases are serious medical conditions that require a combination of conventional treatments such as chemotherapy, radiation therapy, and stem cell transplants. While these treatments are essential in managing the symptoms and fighting the disease, it is also crucial to consider the importance of lifestyle in healing.

A healthy lifestyle can significantly impact the effectiveness of medical treatments and improve

the overall well-being of patients with leukaemia
and blood diseases. Here are some reasons why:

- Reducing Stress: Stress can weaken the
  immune system, making it harder for the
  body to fight off infections and diseases.
  Patients with leukaemia and blood diseases
  are already under a lot of stress due to their
  diagnosis, treatment, and potential side
  effects. Practising stress-reducing
  techniques such as meditation, yoga, or
  deep breathing exercises can help reduce
  stress levels and improve the patient's
  overall health.

- Eating a Healthy Diet: A balanced diet rich
  in vitamins, minerals, and antioxidants can
  help support the body during treatment.
  Patients should aim to eat plenty of fruits,
  vegetables, whole grains, and lean proteins
  while avoiding processed foods and
  excessive amounts of sugar and saturated
  fats. A healthy diet can also help manage
  any side effects from treatment such as
  nausea or fatigue.

- Exercise: Regular exercise can help
  improve cardiovascular health, strengthen
  muscles, and boost energy levels. However,
  it is essential to consult with a healthcare
  provider before starting any new exercise
  routine as some treatments may make

certain activities more challenging or dangerous. Low-impact exercises such as walking or swimming may be more suitable for patients during treatment.

- Getting Enough Sleep: Sleep is crucial for overall health and well-being, especially during treatment for leukaemia and blood diseases. Patients should aim to get at least 7-8 hours of sleep each night to help their bodies rest and recover. Sleep deprivation can weaken the immune system and increase stress levels, making it harder for the body to fight off infections and diseases.

- Quitting Smoking: Smoking can weaken the immune system and increase the risk of complications during treatment for leukaemia and blood diseases. Quitting smoking is essential for improving overall health and reducing the risk of developing secondary cancers or other health problems related to smoking.

In conclusion, a healthy lifestyle is crucial for patients with leukaemia and blood diseases during treatment. By reducing stress, eating a healthy diet, exercising regularly, getting enough sleep, and quitting smoking, patients can improve their overall health and well-being while supporting their bodies during treatment. It is essential to consult with a healthcare provider before making any significant lifestyle changes to ensure they are safe and appropriate for the patient's specific situation.

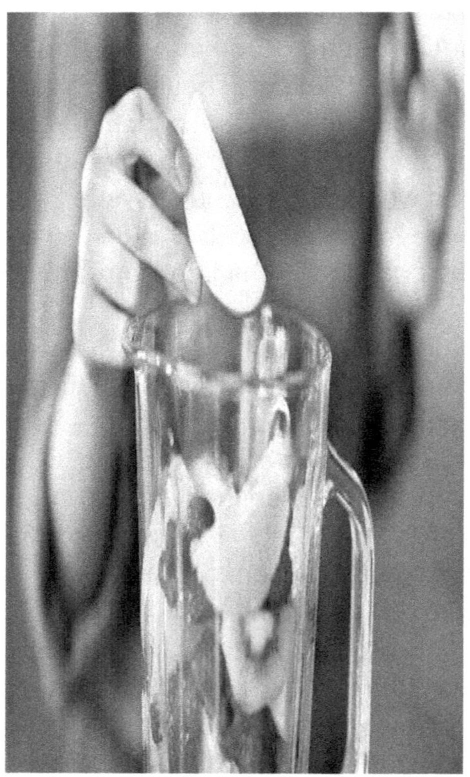

CHAPTER ONE

Understanding Leukaemia

Leukaemia is a form of cancer that affects the blood and bone marrow, which is the spongy tissue inside bones that produces blood cells. Unlike other types of cancer, leukaemia involves the uncontrolled growth and accumulation of abnormal white blood cells, which can crowd out normal cells and disrupt the body's ability to fight infections and control bleeding.

There are several types of leukaemia, classified based on the type of white blood cell affected and the speed of progression. Acute leukaemia, which is more common in children, progresses rapidly and requires immediate treatment. Chronic leukaemia, which is more common in adults, progresses more slowly but may require long-term management.

In acute leukaemia, the abnormal white blood cells are not fully developed and cannot function properly. This can lead to a variety of symptoms, including fever, fatigue, weakness, easy bruising or bleeding, bone pain, and swollen lymph nodes or liver. In chronic leukaemia, the abnormal white blood cells are more mature but still unable to function properly, leading to symptoms such as fatigue, weakness, weight loss, night sweats, and frequent infections.

The exact causes of leukaemia are not fully understood, but it is believed to result from a combination of genetic and environmental factors. Some people may be born with mutations that increase their risk of developing leukaemia, while others may develop mutations later in life due to exposure to certain chemicals or radiation.

Treatment for leukaemia typically involves a combination of chemotherapy, radiation therapy, targeted therapy (which uses drugs that specifically target the abnormal cells), stem cell transplantation (which replaces damaged bone marrow with healthy stem cells), and supportive care (which aims to manage symptoms and side effects). The specific treatment plan will depend on several factors, including the type and stage of leukaemia, the patient's age and overall health, and the preferences of the patient and their healthcare team.

Leukaemia is a complex disease that affects the production and function of white blood cells in the body. While there is still much to learn about its causes and treatment, advances in research and technology are helping to improve outcomes for patients with this challenging condition. By continuing to study leukaemia and develop new treatments and strategies for prevention and management, we can work towards a brighter future for those affected by this disease.

Types and Subtypes

Leukaemia is a type of cancer that affects the blood-forming cells in the bone marrow. These cells, known as hematopoietic stem cells, give rise to three main types of blood cells: red blood cells, white blood cells, and platelets. In leukaemia, there is an uncontrolled proliferation of abnormal white blood cells, which interfere with the production and function of normal blood cells.

There are several types of leukaemia, classified based on the type of white blood cell affected and the rate at which the disease progresses. Acute leukaemia and chronic leukaemia are the two basic types of leukemia. Acute leukaemia is characterised by a rapid onset and progression of symptoms, while chronic leukaemia develops more slowly over time.

Acute Leukaemia:

Acute myeloid leukaemia (AML) is a type of acute leukaemia that affects myeloid cells, which give rise to red blood cells, platelets, and some types of white blood cells. AML is characterised by the accumulation of immature myeloid cells in the bone marrow and peripheral blood, leading to a decrease in the production of normal blood cells.

Acute lymphoblastic leukaemia (ALL) is a type of acute leukaemia that affects lymphoid cells, which give rise to white blood cells called lymphocytes. ALL is characterised by the accumulation of immature lymphoid cells in the bone marrow and peripheral blood, leading to a decrease in the production of normal lymphocytes.

Chronic Leukaemia:

Chronic myeloid leukaemia (CML) is a type of chronic leukaemia that affects myeloid cells. CML is characterised by the accumulation of mature but abnormal myeloid cells in the bone marrow and peripheral blood, leading to an increase in the number of white blood cells.

Chronic lymphocytic leukaemia (CLL) is a type of chronic leukaemia that affects lymphoid cells. CLL is characterised by the accumulation of mature but abnormal lymphocytes in the bone marrow and peripheral blood, leading to an increase in the number of white blood cells.

Subtypes:

Within each type of leukaemia, there are several subtypes based on genetic mutations and other characteristics. For example, AML can be further classified into subtypes based on genetic mutations such as FLT3-ITD or NPM1-mutated. ALL can be further classified into subtypes based on the expression of certain proteins such as CD19 or CD20. CML can be further classified into subtypes based on genetic mutations such as BCR-ABL or Ph+ chromosomes. CLL can be further classified into subtypes based on genetic mutations such as 17p deletion or 11q23 rearrangement. Understanding these subtypes can help guide treatment decisions and prognosticate outcomes for patients with leukaemia.

Causes and Risk Factors

Leukaemia is a type of cancer that affects the blood and bone marrow, leading to the uncontrolled growth of abnormal white blood cells. While the exact causes of leukaemia are not fully understood, several factors have been identified that increase the risk of developing this disease.

- Genetic Factors: Some people may inherit genetic mutations that increase their risk of leukaemia. For example, mutations in genes such as FLT3, CEBPA, and RUNX1 have been linked to an increased risk of acute myeloid leukaemia (AML).

- Environmental Factors: Exposure to certain environmental factors can increase the risk of leukaemia. For example, exposure to ionising radiation, such as that found in high-dose radiation therapy or nuclear accidents, can increase the risk of developing leukaemia. Additionally, exposure to certain chemicals, such as benzene and pesticides, has been linked to an increased risk of leukaemia.

- Viral Infections: Certain viruses, such as human T-cell lymphotropic virus (HTLV) and human immunodeficiency virus (HIV), have been linked to an increased risk of leukaemia. Infected individuals may develop leukaemia as a result of the virus damaging their immune system or causing genetic mutations in their cells.

- Medical Treatments: Some medical treatments can increase the risk of developing leukaemia. For example, chemotherapy and radiation therapy used to treat other types of cancer can damage healthy cells in the bone marrow, leading to the development of leukaemia. Additionally, some medications used to treat autoimmune diseases and other conditions can increase the risk of developing leukaemia.

- Age: The risk of developing leukaemia increases with age, with most cases occurring in individuals over the age of 65. This may be due to a combination of genetic and environmental factors that accumulate over time.

In conclusion, while the causes of leukaemia are complex and multifactorial, several factors have been identified that increase the risk of developing this disease. Understanding these causes and risk factors is important for developing strategies for prevention and early detection of leukaemia. Additionally, ongoing research into the genetics and biology of leukaemia is helping to improve our understanding of this disease and develop more effective treatments for those affected by it.

Diagnosis and Staging

Leukaemia is a type of cancer that affects the blood and bone marrow, causing an overproduction of abnormal white blood cells. The diagnosis and staging of leukaemia are crucial steps in understanding the disease, as they provide information about the type, severity, and spread of the cancer. In this article, we will discuss the diagnosis and staging of leukaemia.

Diagnosis:

The diagnosis of leukaemia involves several tests to confirm the presence of cancerous cells in the blood and bone marrow. Some of the common diagnostic tests for leukaemia include:

1. Complete Blood Count (CBC): This test measures the number and type of cells in the blood, including white blood cells, red blood cells, and platelets. In leukaemia, there is an abnormal increase in white blood cells.

2. Bone Marrow Aspiration and Biopsy: This procedure involves removing a small amount of bone marrow from the hip or pelvic bone using a needle. The sample is then examined under a microscope to check for the presence of cancerous cells.

3. Cytogenetic Analysis: This test examines the chromosomes in the cancerous cells to identify any abnormalities or changes that may help in determining the type and subtype of leukaemia.

4. Fluorescence In Situ Hybridization (FISH): This test uses fluorescent dyes to identify specific genetic changes or abnormalities in the cancerous cells.

5. Immunophenotyping: This test uses antibodies to identify specific proteins on the surface of white blood cells to determine their type and maturity level.

Once leukaemia is diagnosed, it is staged to determine its severity and spread. The staging system used for leukaemia is called the French-American-British (FAB) system or the World Health Organization (WHO) classification system. The stages are as follows:

1. Chronic Phase: This is the initial stage of leukaemia, where there are a large number of abnormal white blood cells in the bone marrow but not in the bloodstream. Symptoms may be mild or absent during this phase.

2. Accelerated Phase: This stage is characterised by an increase in blast cells (immature white blood cells) in the bone marrow and bloodstream, indicating that the disease is progressing rapidly. Symptoms may include fever, fatigue, and weight loss.

3. Blast Crisis/Acute Leukaemia: This stage is marked by a rapid increase in blast cells in both the bone marrow and bloodstream, leading to severe symptoms such as fever, bleeding, and organ failure. This stage requires immediate treatment as it is considered an emergency medical condition.

In conclusion, understanding the diagnosis and staging of leukaemia is crucial for developing an effective treatment plan for patients with this disease. Early detection and prompt treatment can improve outcomes and increase survival rates for individuals with leukaemia.

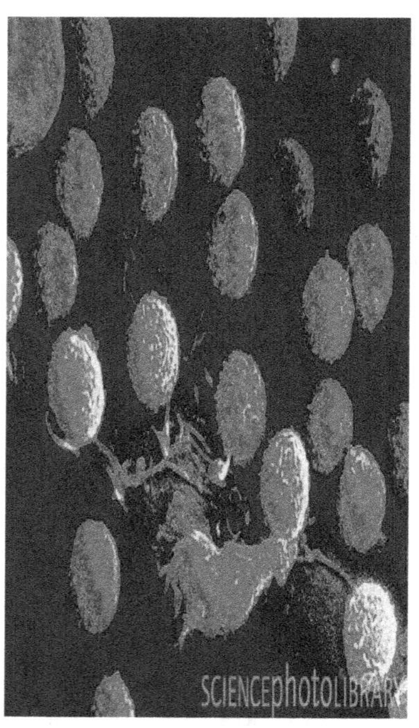

CHAPTER TWO

Treatment Approaches

Conventional Treatments

Leukaemia and other blood diseases are complex medical conditions that require comprehensive treatment approaches. While advancements in modern medicine have led to the development of innovative therapies, conventional treatments remain a critical part of the treatment landscape. In this article, we will explore conventional treatments in the context of leukaemia and blood diseases.

Chemotherapy

Chemotherapy is a conventional treatment that involves the use of drugs to destroy cancer cells. It is commonly used to treat leukaemia and other blood diseases. Chemotherapy works by targeting rapidly dividing cells, including cancer cells, which can cause side effects such as hair loss, nausea, and fatigue. The specific chemotherapy drugs used depend on the type and stage of the disease.

Radiation Therapy

Radiation therapy is another conventional treatment that uses high-energy radiation to destroy cancer cells. It is commonly used to treat leukaemia and other blood diseases that have spread to other parts of the body. Radiation therapy can be delivered externally or internally, depending on the location and extent of the disease. External radiation therapy involves the use of a machine to deliver radiation beams to the affected area, while internal radiation therapy involves the use of radioactive materials placed directly into the body.

Stem Cell Transplantation

Stem cell transplantation is a conventional treatment that involves replacing damaged or diseased stem cells with healthy ones. Stem cells are immature cells that can develop into different types of cells in the body, including blood cells. Stem cell transplantation is commonly used to treat leukaemia and other blood diseases that have not responded to other treatments or have relapsed. The procedure involves collecting stem cells from a donor or from the patient's own body, cleaning them, and infusing them back into the patient's bloodstream.

Immunotherapy

Immunotherapy is a conventional treatment that involves using the patient's own immune system to fight cancer cells. It works by either stimulating the immune system to attack cancer cells or by using antibodies or other immune system components to directly target cancer cells. Immunotherapy is commonly used to treat leukaemia and other blood diseases that have not responded to other treatments or have relapsed. The specific immunotherapy drugs used depend on the type and stage of the disease

In conclusion, conventional treatments such as chemotherapy, radiation therapy, stem cell transplantation, and immunotherapy remain critical components of treatment approaches for leukaemia and other blood diseases. While advancements in modern medicine have led to the development of innovative therapies, these conventional treatments continue to provide effective options for patients with these complex medical conditions. The choice of treatment depends on several factors, including the type and stage of the disease, patient age and overall health, and potential side effects of each treatment option. It is essential for healthcare providers to work closely with patients to develop personalised treatment plans that consider all these factors.

Complementary and Alternative Therapies

Leukaemia and other blood diseases are complex medical conditions that require a multidisciplinary approach to treatment. While conventional therapies such as chemotherapy, radiation therapy, and stem cell transplantation are the primary treatment options, complementary and alternative therapies (CAM) are increasingly being explored as adjunctive or alternative approaches. In this article, we will discuss some of the CAM therapies that have shown promise in the treatment of leukaemia and blood diseases.

1. Acupuncture: Acupuncture is a traditional Chinese medicine (TCM) technique that involves inserting thin needles into specific points on the body to stimulate healing and reduce pain. Some studies have suggested that acupuncture may help alleviate symptoms associated with leukaemia treatment such as fatigue, nausea, and pain. A randomised controlled trial published in the Journal of Clinical Oncology found that acupuncture significantly reduced chemotherapy-induced nausea and vomiting in patients with acute myeloid leukaemia (AML).

2. Herbal Medicine: Herbal medicine is a form of CAM that involves using plant-based remedies to treat various health conditions. Some herbs have been shown to have anticancer properties and may be beneficial in the treatment of leukaemia. For example, curcumin, a compound found in turmeric, has been shown to have anti-leukemic effects in preclinical studies. A phase II clinical trial published in the Journal of Clinical Oncology found that curcumin combined with chemotherapy improved overall response rates in patients with AML.

3. *Mind-Body Therapies:* Mind-body therapies such as meditation, yoga, and relaxation techniques are used to promote relaxation, reduce stress, and improve overall well-being. These therapies may also have beneficial effects on leukaemia patients by reducing anxiety and depression, which are common psychological issues associated with cancer diagnosis and treatment. A randomised controlled trial published in the Journal of Psychosocial Oncology found that mindfulness meditation significantly reduced anxiety and depression symptoms in patients with chronic lymphocytic leukaemia (CLL).

4. *Nutritional Therapies:* Nutritional therapies involve using dietary modifications to improve overall health and well-being. Some dietary supplements such as vitamin C and vitamin E have been shown to have anticancer properties and may be beneficial in the treatment of leukaemia. A randomised controlled trial published in the Journal of Clinical Oncology found that vitamin C combined with chemotherapy improved overall response rates in patients with AML.

5. *Traditional Chinese Medicine (TCM):* TCM is a holistic medical system that combines various modalities such as acupuncture, herbal medicine, massage therapy, and meditation to treat various health conditions. TCM has been used for centuries to treat cancer patients in China, and some studies have suggested that TCM may have beneficial effects on leukaemia patients by improving overall well-being and reducing side effects associated with conventional treatments. A systematic review published in the Journal of Traditional Chinese Medicine found that TCM significantly improved quality of life and reduced fatigue in patients with CLL undergoing chemotherapy.

In conclusion, CAM therapies such as acupuncture, herbal medicine, mind-body therapies, nutritional therapies, and TCM are increasingly being explored as adjunctive or alternative approaches to conventional treatments for leukaemia and blood diseases. While some studies have suggested promising results, more research is needed to fully understand the safety and efficacy of these therapies. Patients should consult their healthcare providers before incorporating any CAM therapies into their treatment plans to ensure they are safe and appropriate for their specific condition.

Integrative Medicine

Integrative medicine is a comprehensive approach to healthcare that incorporates conventional medical treatments as well as complementary and alternative therapies. This approach has gained popularity in recent years, particularly in the treatment of chronic diseases such as leukaemia and blood disorders.

Leukaemia is a type of cancer that affects the blood-forming cells in the bone marrow. Conventional treatments for leukaemia include chemotherapy, radiation therapy, and stem cell transplantation. While these treatments can be effective, they also have significant side effects, such as nausea, fatigue, and hair loss.

Integrative medicine offers additional therapies that can help manage these side effects and improve overall well-being. Some of these therapies include acupuncture, meditation, and yoga. Acupuncture can help relieve pain and reduce stress, while meditation and yoga can help manage anxiety and improve relaxation.

Acupuncture is a technique that includes inserting small needles into certain places on the body in order to promote the body's natural healing mechanisms. Studies have shown that acupuncture can help reduce chemotherapy-induced nausea and vomiting, as well as improve overall quality of life for leukaemia patients (1).

Meditation involves focusing the mind on a specific thought or object to achieve a state of relaxation and mental clarity. Meditation has been shown to help reduce stress and anxiety, which can be beneficial for leukaemia patients undergoing intensive treatments (2).

Yoga combines physical postures, breathing exercises, and meditation to promote overall health and well-being. Yoga has been shown to help improve flexibility, strength, and balance, as well as reduce stress and anxiety (3).

In addition to these therapies, integrative medicine also includes dietary supplements and herbal remedies that may have anti-cancer properties. For example, turmeric, a spice commonly used in Indian cuisine, contains a compound called curcumin that has been shown to have anti-inflammatory and anti-cancer properties (4).

While integrative medicine offers many benefits for leukaemia patients, it's important to remember that these therapies should be used in conjunction with conventional medical treatments. Patients should always consult with their healthcare provider before starting any new therapy or supplement regimen.

In conclusion, integrative medicine offers a holistic approach to healthcare that combines conventional medical treatments with complementary and alternative therapies. For leukaemia patients undergoing intensive treatments, integrative therapies such as acupuncture, meditation, yoga, and dietary supplements can help manage side effects and improve overall well-being. However, it's important to remember that these therapies should be used in conjunction with conventional medical treatments under the guidance of a healthcare provider. By taking a holistic approach to healthcare, we can provide our patients with the best possible outcomes for their treatment journey.

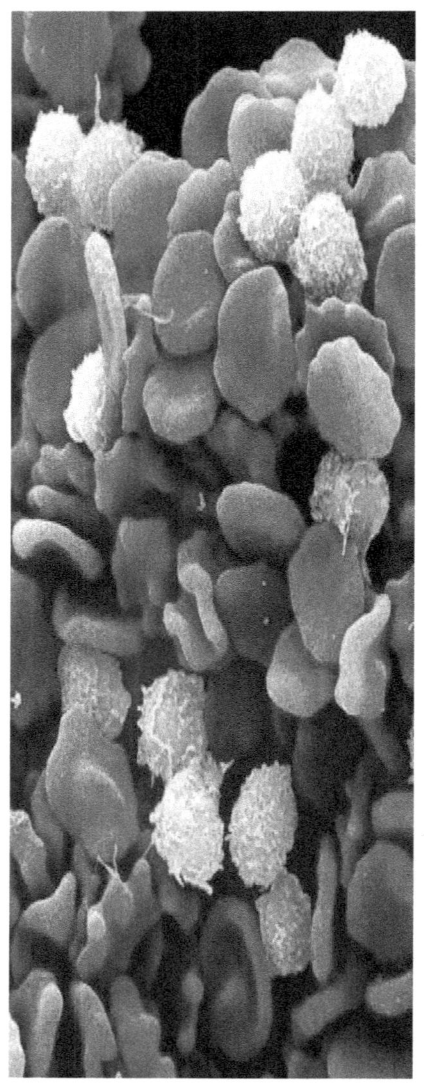

CHAPTER THREE

Nutrition for Recovery

Building a Nutrient-Rich Plate

Leukaemia and other blood diseases can take a significant toll on the body, making it crucial for individuals undergoing treatment to prioritise a nutrient-rich diet for recovery. A nutrient-rich plate is essential to support the body's healing process, boost energy levels, and manage any potential side effects of treatment. In this article, we will discuss some key elements to consider when building a nutrient-rich plate for individuals with leukaemia and blood diseases.

1. Protein:

Protein is essential for building and repairing tissues, including those affected by leukaemia or blood diseases. Good sources of protein include lean meats, poultry, fish, beans, lentils, and tofu. Every day, aim for 1-1.5 grams of protein per kilogram of body weight.

2. Fruits and Vegetables:

Fruits and vegetables are rich in vitamins, minerals, and antioxidants that support overall health and help combat the effects of chemotherapy or radiation therapy. Choose a variety of colours to ensure a range of nutrients. Make an effort to consume at least five servings per day.

3. Whole Grains:

Whole grains are an excellent source of fibre, which can help prevent constipation, a common side effect of treatment. Choose whole-grain bread, pasta, rice, and cereal instead of refined grains.

4. Healthy Fats:

Healthy fats such as those found in avocados, nuts, seeds, and olive oil can help absorb fat-soluble vitamins like vitamin A and D. Limit your intake of saturated and trans fats found in processed foods and fried foods.

5. Hydration:

Staying hydrated is essential for overall health and can help prevent constipation caused by treatment. Drink plenty of water throughout the day and limit caffeinated beverages that can dehydrate the body.

6. Consult with a Registered Dietitian:

A registered dietitian can provide personalised guidance on nutrition during treatment based on individual needs and preferences. They can also offer strategies to manage any potential side effects of treatment such as nausea or loss of appetite.

In summary, building a nutrient-rich plate for individuals with leukaemia or blood diseases should include protein-rich foods such as lean meats, poultry, fish, beans, lentils, and tofu; fruits and vegetables; whole grains; healthy fats; hydration; and consultation with a registered dietitian for personalised guidance. By prioritising a nutrient-rich diet during treatment, individuals can support their bodies' healing process and manage any potential side effects more effectively.

Anti-Cancer Foods

Leukaemia and other blood diseases are types of cancer that affect the blood-forming cells in the body. While traditional cancer treatments such as chemotherapy and radiation therapy are essential in managing these conditions, nutrition also plays a crucial role in supporting recovery. In this article, we will explore some anti-cancer foods that can help individuals with leukaemia and blood diseases in their nutrition for recovery.

- Berries: Berries such as strawberries, blueberries, raspberries, and blackberries are rich in antioxidants called anthocyanins. These antioxidants have been shown to have anti-cancer properties by preventing the growth and spread of cancer cells. Additionally, berries contain fibre, which can help promote a healthy digestive system and prevent constipation, a common side effect of chemotherapy.

☐ Leafy Greens: Leafy greens such as spinach, kale, and collard greens are packed with vitamins and minerals that are essential for overall health. They are also rich in antioxidants called carotenoids, which have been shown to have anti-cancer properties by preventing the growth and spread of cancer cells. Additionally, leafy greens contain fibre, which can help promote a healthy digestive system and prevent constipation.

☐ Citrus Fruits: Citrus fruits such as oranges, lemons, limes, and grapefruits are rich in vitamin C, which is a powerful antioxidant that can help prevent the formation of cancer cells. Additionally, citrus fruits contain flavonoids, which are compounds that have been shown to have anti-cancer properties by preventing the growth and spread of cancer cells.

☐ Garlic: Garlic is a pungent herb that has been used for centuries for its medicinal properties. It contains compounds called allicin and sulphur compounds that have been shown to have anti-cancer properties by preventing the growth and spread of cancer cells. Additionally, garlic has immune-boosting properties that can help support the body's natural defence system against cancer cells.

- [ ] Turmeric: Turmeric is a spice that is often used in Indian cuisine. It contains a compound called curcumin, which has been shown to have anti-cancer properties by preventing the growth and spread of cancer cells. Additionally, turmeric has anti-inflammatory properties that can help reduce inflammation in the body, which is associated with an increased risk of cancer.

- [ ] Green Tea: Green tea is rich in antioxidants called catechins, which have been shown to have anti-cancer properties by preventing the growth and spread of cancer cells. Additionally, green tea contains caffeine and L-theanine, which can help promote relaxation and reduce stress levels, both of which are important for overall health and wellbeing during recovery from leukaemia or blood diseases.

In conclusion, incorporating these anti-cancer foods into one's diet can provide numerous health benefits during recovery from leukaemia or blood diseases. It is essential to work with a healthcare provider or a registered dietitian to develop a personalised nutrition plan that meets one's specific needs during treatment and recovery. By making healthy food choices and working closely with healthcare providers, individuals with leukaemia or blood diseases can improve their overall health and wellbeing during this challenging time.

Meal Planning Tips

Meal planning is a crucial aspect of nutrition for individuals undergoing treatment for leukaemia and blood diseases. Proper nutrition can help manage symptoms, support the body during treatment, and promote overall health. Here are some meal planning tips for individuals with leukaemia and blood diseases:

1. Consult with a registered dietitian: A registered dietitian can provide personalised nutrition advice based on your specific condition, treatment plan, and dietary preferences. They can also help you address any nutritional deficiencies or concerns that may arise during treatment.

2. Focus on whole foods: Choose whole, nutrient-dense foods such as fruits, vegetables, whole grains, and lean proteins. These foods provide essential vitamins, minerals, and antioxidants that can help support the body during treatment.

3. Incorporate protein-rich foods: Protein is essential for building and repairing cells, which is important during treatment when the body may be undergoing damage. Good sources of protein include lean meats, poultry, fish, beans, and lentils.

4. Stay hydrated: Dehydration is common during treatment due to increased urination and vomiting. Drink plenty of water throughout the day to stay hydrated and avoid dehydration-related symptoms such as dizziness and fatigue.

5. Manage side effects: Treatment for leukaemia and blood diseases can cause side effects such as nausea, vomiting, and mouth sores. To manage these symptoms, choose soft, easy-to-swallow foods such as soups, pureed fruits, and smoothies. Avoid spicy or acidic foods that can irritate the mouth or stomach.

6. Limit processed foods: Processed foods are often high in sugar, salt, and unhealthy fats that can negatively impact overall health. Instead, focus on whole foods that are minimally processed to ensure optimal nutrition.

7. Plan ahead: Meal planning can help ensure that you have healthy options available when you don't feel like cooking or grocery shopping. Plan meals for the week ahead of time and prepare meals in advance to make healthy eating easier during busy times.

<u>**8. _Practise mindful eating:_**</u> Eating mindfully can help you enjoy your meals more fully and make healthier choices. Take time to savour each bite, chew your food thoroughly, and listen to your body's hunger and fullness cues to avoid overeating or undereating.

By following these meal planning tips, individuals with leukaemia and blood diseases can support their bodies during treatment while promoting overall health and wellbeing.

CHAPTER FOUR

The Healing Power of Juicing

Juices for Strength and Recovery

Juices have gained immense popularity in recent years as a healthy and refreshing alternative to sugary drinks. However, their benefits go beyond just hydration and taste. Juices can also be incredibly beneficial for individuals undergoing treatment for leukaemia and other blood diseases. In this article, we will explore the healing power of juicing and the specific juices that can help with strength and recovery during cancer treatment.

Leukaemia is a type of cancer that affects the blood-forming cells in the bone marrow. Treatment for leukaemia often involves chemotherapy, radiation therapy, or a bone marrow transplant. These treatments can be incredibly taxing on the body, leading to fatigue, weakness, and nutrient deficiencies. This is where juicing comes in.

Juices are packed with vitamins, minerals, and antioxidants that can help support the body during cancer treatment. They are also easy to digest and absorb, making them an ideal choice for individuals experiencing nausea or digestive issues. Here are some of the best juices for strength and recovery during cancer treatment:

- Carrot Juice: Carrots are high in beta-carotene, which the body converts to vitamin A. Vitamin A is essential for maintaining healthy skin, mucous membranes, and vision. It also has anti-inflammatory properties that can help reduce inflammation in the body. Carrot juice is also high in potassium, which can help regulate blood pressure and prevent muscle cramps.

- Beet Juice: Beets are rich in folate, which is important for cell growth and division. They are also high in antioxidants like betaine and betacyanin, which have been shown to have anti-inflammatory and anti-cancer properties. Beet juice is also rich in iron, which can help prevent anaemia, a common side effect of chemotherapy.

- Ginger Juice: Ginger has anti-inflammatory and anti-nausea properties that can help alleviate some of the side effects of chemotherapy, such as nausea and vomiting. It also has anti-cancer properties and may help prevent the spread of cancer cells.

- Spinach Juice: Spinach is rich in iron, vitamin K, and vitamin C. Iron is important for preventing anaemia, while vitamin K is important for blood clotting and bone health. Vitamin C is an antioxidant that can help protect the body from damage caused by free radicals.

- Celery Juice: Celery is rich in potassium, magnesium, and vitamin K. Potassium is important for maintaining healthy blood pressure, while magnesium is important for bone health and preventing muscle cramps. Vitamin K is important for blood clotting and preventing bruising.

In addition to these juices, it's also important to include other healthy foods in your diet during cancer treatment. Some good options include:

1. Lean protein sources like chicken, fish, and beans to help build muscle mass and prevent weight loss.
2. Whole grains like brown rice, quinoa, and whole wheat bread provide complex carbohydrates for energy.
3. Fruits like berries, citrus fruits, and melons provide vitamins and minerals like vitamin C and potassium.
4. Nuts and seeds like almonds, chia seeds, and flax seeds provide healthy fats and protein.

5. Herbal teas like ginger tea or peppermint tea to help alleviate nausea or digestive issues caused by chemotherapy or radiation therapy.

In conclusion, juicing can be a powerful tool for supporting the body during cancer treatment. The specific juices recommended here are just a few examples of the many options available - it's always best to consult with a healthcare provider or a registered dietitian to determine which juices are best for your individual needs during treatment for leukaemia or other blood diseases. By incorporating a variety of healthy foods into your diet along with these recommended juices, you can help support your body's strength and recovery during this challenging time.

Juicing Recipes

Juicing has gained popularity in recent years as a healthy and convenient way to consume fruits and vegetables. However, for individuals suffering from leukaemia and blood diseases, juicing can have a powerful healing effect. In this article, we will explore some juicing recipes that are specifically beneficial for those with these conditions and the science behind their healing properties.

Leukaemia is a type of cancer that affects the blood-forming cells in the bone marrow. It can lead to an overproduction of abnormal white blood cells, which can interfere with the production of healthy red blood cells and platelets. which can crowd out healthy cells and impair the body's ability to fight infection.This can result in symptoms such as fatigue, weakness, and easy bruising or bleeding. Blood disorders, on the other hand, refer to a range of conditions that affect the production, function, or circulation of blood cells.

Blood diseases, such as sickle cell anaemia and thalassemia, also affect the production of red blood cells, leading to symptoms such as fatigue, shortness of breath, and jaundice.

While conventional medical treatments such as chemotherapy and radiation therapy are often necessary for managing leukaemia and blood disorders, complementary therapies such as juicing can also provide significant benefits. Juicing allows for the consumption of large quantities of nutrient-dense fruits and vegetables in a convenient and easily digestible form, providing the body with essential vitamins, minerals, and antioxidants that can help support overall health and wellbeing.

Juicing can help alleviate some of these symptoms by providing a concentrated source of nutrients that are easily absorbed by the body. Here are some juicing recipes that are particularly beneficial for individuals with leukaemia and blood diseases:

1. Beetroot and Carrot Juice:

Beetroot is rich in betaine, a compound that helps reduce inflammation and protects against oxidative stress. It also contains betacyanins, which have been shown to have anticancer properties. Carrots are high in beta-carotene, which is converted into vitamin A in the body and helps boost the immune system. This juice is also rich in potassium, which helps regulate blood pressure and prevent fluid buildup in the body.

Ingredients:
- 2 medium beetroots
- 4 medium carrots
- 1 inch ginger root (optional)
- 1 lemon (optional)
- Water (as needed)

Instructions:
1. Wash all ingredients thoroughly.
2. Cut beetroot and carrots into small pieces.
3. Add beetroot, carrots, ginger root (if using), and lemon juice (if using) into a juicer.
4. Add water as needed to achieve desired consistency.
5. Stir well before drinking.
6. Drink immediately for best results.

2. Spinach and Apple Juice:

Spinach is rich in iron, which is essential for individuals with blood diseases such as sickle cell anaemia or thalassemia who may have low iron levels due to reduced red blood cell production. Apples are high in fibre and vitamin C, which helps boost the immune system and promote healthy digestion. This juice is also rich in antioxidants such as vitamin A and vitamin C, which help protect against oxidative stress and inflammation.

Ingredients:
- 2 cups spinach leaves
- 2 medium apples (preferably green apples)
- Water (as needed)

Instructions:
1. Wash all ingredients thoroughly.
2. Cut apples into small pieces.
3. Add spinach leaves and apples into a juicer.
4. Add water as needed to achieve desired consistency.
5. Stir well before drinking.
6. Drink immediately for best results.

3. Ginger Turmeric Tonic:

- 1 inch fresh ginger root
- 1/2 lemon, peeled
- 1/2 cucumber
- 1/2 apple
- 1/2 inch fresh turmeric root
- 1/2 cup water

Ginger and turmeric are both powerful anti-inflammatory agents that can help reduce inflammation in the body, which is often elevated in individuals with leukaemia and blood disorders. Lemon is rich in vitamin C, which can help support the immune system, while cucumber and apple provide hydration and fibre. This tonic is best consumed first thing in the morning on an empty stomach.

4. Beetroot Carrot Juice:

- 2 medium beetroots
- 4 medium carrots
- 1 orange
- 1 lemon, peeled
- 1 inch fresh ginger root
- 1/2 cup water

Beetroots are rich in betaine, a compound that has been found to have anti-cancer properties. Carrots are high in beta-carotene, which can help support healthy vision and skin. Oranges and lemons are both rich in vitamin C, while ginger adds a spicy kick that can help stimulate digestion and reduce inflammation. This juice is best consumed mid-morning or mid-afternoon as a snack or light meal replacement.

5. Kale Spinach Green Juice:

- 1 bunch kale (stems removed)
- 1 bunch spinach (stems removed)
- 1 cucumber
- 1 apple (cored)
- 1 lemon, peeled
- 1 inch fresh ginger root
- 1/2 cup water

Kale and spinach are both rich in chlorophyll, which can help support healthy blood cell production. Cucumber provides hydration, while apple adds sweetness. Lemon adds a tangy flavour and helps alkalize the body's pH level. Ginger adds a spicy kick that can help stimulate digestion and reduce inflammation. This juice is best consumed midday as a light meal replacement or snack.

In addition to these recipes, it's also important to note that individuals with leukaemia or blood disorders should consult with their healthcare provider before starting any new dietary or supplement regimen to ensure it does not interfere with their treatment plan or medication regimen. While juicing can provide significant benefits when used as part of a holistic approach to health and wellness, it should not be used as a substitute for conventional medical treatments or as a means of delaying or avoiding necessary medical care.

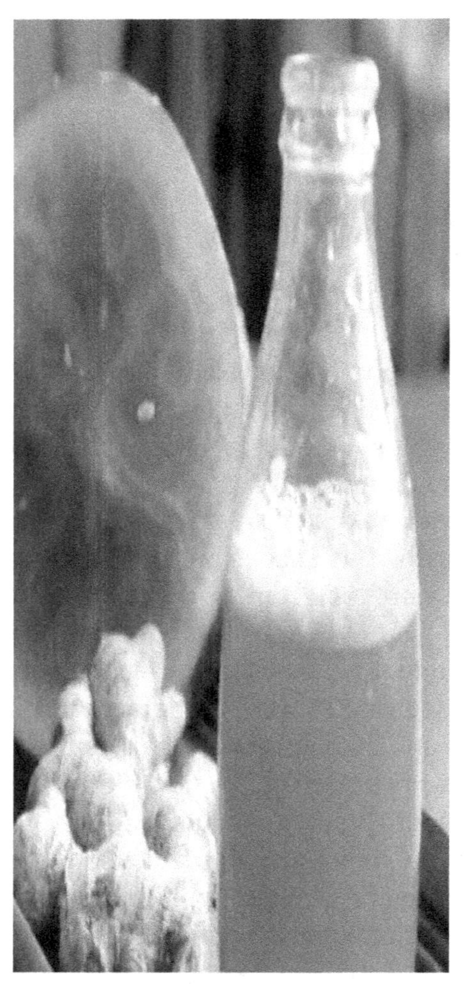

CHAPTER FIVE

Lifestyle Optimisation

Exercise and Movement

Exercise and movement play a crucial role in lifestyle optimization for individuals with leukaemia and blood diseases. While these conditions can be debilitating and often require intensive medical treatment, incorporating regular physical activity into one's routine can have numerous benefits for overall health and well-being.

Firstly, exercise can help to manage symptoms associated with leukaemia and blood diseases. For example, regular aerobic activity has been shown to reduce fatigue, a common symptom experienced by many individuals with these conditions. Exercise also helps to improve cardiovascular health, which is particularly important for individuals with leukaemia as they may be at higher risk of developing heart problems due to the effects of chemotherapy and other treatments.

Secondly, exercise can help to strengthen muscles and improve bone density, which is important for individuals with blood diseases such as myeloma or multiple myeloma. These conditions can lead to bone loss and fractures, making regular exercise an essential part of managing the condition and reducing the risk of further complications.

Thirdly, exercise can help to boost the immune system, which is particularly important for individuals with leukaemia or other blood diseases as they may be more susceptible to infections due to the effects of chemotherapy or other treatments. Regular exercise has been shown to increase the production of white blood cells, which are responsible for fighting off infection.

Finally, exercise can help to improve overall quality of life for individuals with leukaemia and blood diseases. Regular physical activity has been shown to reduce stress, anxiety, and depression, all of which are common concerns for individuals undergoing treatment for these conditions. Exercise also provides a sense of control and empowerment, helping individuals to feel more in charge of their health and well-being.

Of course, it's important to note that individuals with leukaemia or blood diseases should always consult with their healthcare provider before starting any new exercise program. Some treatments may make certain types of exercise more challenging or risky, and it's essential to ensure that any exercise program is tailored to individual needs and abilities.

In summary, incorporating regular exercise and movement into one's lifestyle is an essential part of optimising health and well-being for individuals with leukaemia and blood diseases. By managing symptoms, improving cardiovascular health, boosting the immune system, and enhancing overall quality of life, exercise provides a powerful tool for managing these conditions and improving outcomes for affected individuals.

Stress Management

Stress is a common experience for individuals dealing with chronic illnesses such as leukaemia and blood diseases. While medical treatments and therapies are crucial in managing these conditions, it's equally essential to prioritise stress management as part of a holistic approach to lifestyle optimization. Stress can have detrimental effects on physical and mental health, exacerbating symptoms and hindering recovery. In this article, we'll explore practical strategies for managing stress in individuals with leukaemia and blood diseases.

1. Mindfulness Meditation: Mindfulness meditation is a technique that involves focusing one's attention on the present moment, accepting thoughts and feelings without judgement. This practice can help individuals develop greater self-awareness, reduce anxiety, and improve overall well-being. Studies have shown that mindfulness meditation can also enhance immune function, which is particularly beneficial for individuals with leukaemia and blood diseases.

2. Exercise: Regular exercise is essential for maintaining overall health and reducing stress levels. Exercise releases endorphins, which are natural mood boosters, and can help individuals feel more positive and energised. Gentle exercises such as yoga, Pilates, or swimming can be particularly beneficial for individuals with leukaemia or blood diseases as they are low-impact and help to build strength and flexibility.

3. Relaxation Techniques: Relaxation techniques such as deep breathing, progressive muscle relaxation, and guided imagery can help individuals manage stress levels by promoting relaxation and reducing tension in the body. These techniques can be practised at home or during therapy sessions to help individuals learn how to manage stress in their daily lives.

4. Support Groups: Joining support groups can provide individuals with leukaemia or blood diseases with a sense of community and connection. These groups offer a safe space for individuals to share their experiences, learn coping strategies, and provide emotional support to one another.

5. Healthy Diet: Eating a healthy diet rich in fruits, vegetables, whole grains, and lean proteins can help individuals manage stress levels by providing the body with the nutrients it needs to function optimally. Additionally, avoiding processed foods, caffeine, and alcohol can help reduce stress levels by preventing spikes in blood sugar and promoting relaxation.

6. Cognitive Behavioral Therapy (CBT): CBT is a form of talk therapy that helps individuals identify negative thought patterns and replace them with more positive ones. This therapy can be particularly beneficial for individuals with leukaemia or blood diseases as it helps them develop coping strategies for managing the emotional toll of their condition.

In conclusion, managing stress is an essential component of lifestyle optimization for individuals with leukaemia or blood diseases. By incorporating mindfulness meditation, exercise, relaxation techniques, support groups, healthy diet, and CBT into their daily routines, individuals can learn how to manage stress levels effectively while promoting overall health and well-being. It's essential to work closely with healthcare providers to develop a personalised stress management plan that meets individual needs and circumstances.

Quality Sleep

As someone living with leukaemia or a blood disorder, getting a good night's sleep is crucial for your overall health and wellbeing. Quality sleep is not only essential for your physical health but also plays a significant role in managing the symptoms of these conditions. In this article, we will explore the importance of quality sleep in lifestyle optimisation for leukaemia and blood diseases.

Firstly, let's understand what quality sleep is. It's a state of deep rest that allows your body to repair and regenerate itself. During sleep, your brain processes the events of the day, consolidates memories, and prepares you for the next day's activities. A good night's sleep is typically seven to eight hours long, and you wake up feeling refreshed and energised.

Now let's see how quality sleep can help manage the symptoms of leukaemia and blood disorders:

Reduces Fatigue

Fatigue is a common symptom of leukaemia and blood disorders. Lack of sleep or poor-quality sleep can exacerbate fatigue, making it challenging to carry out daily activities. Getting enough quality sleep can help reduce fatigue and improve energy levels during the day.

Boosts Immune System

Leukaemia and blood disorders weaken the immune system, making it more susceptible to infections. Quality sleep helps boost the immune system by releasing cytokines, which are proteins that help fight infection and inflammation.

Leukaemia and blood disorders can cause emotional distress, leading to anxiety and depression. Quality sleep can help improve mood by reducing stress levels and promoting feelings of calmness and relaxation.

Leukaemia and blood disorders can affect cognitive function, leading to memory loss, confusion, and difficulty concentrating. Quality sleep helps enhance cognitive function by consolidating memories and improving concentration levels.

Leukaemia and blood disorders can cause pain due to bone marrow damage or chemotherapy treatments. Quality sleep helps reduce pain by releasing endorphins, which are natural painkillers produced by the body during sleep.

To optimise your lifestyle for quality sleep while dealing with leukaemia or a blood disorder, here are some tips:

1. Maintain a Sleep Schedule: Every day, even on weekends, go to bed and wake up at the same time. This improves greater sleep quality by regulating your body's internal clock.

2. Create a Sleep-Conducive Environment: Make sure your bedroom is dark, quiet, cool, and comfortable for sleeping. Use blackout curtains or an eye mask to block out light, earplugs to block out noise, and a fan or air conditioner to keep the room cool.

3. Limit Screen Time Before Bed: The blue light emitted by screens can disrupt your body's production of melatonin, a hormone that helps promote sleepiness. Avoid using screens for at least an hour before bedtime or use blue light filters on your devices to minimise the impact on your sleep cycle.

4. Practice Relaxation Techniques: Incorporate relaxation techniques such as meditation, deep breathing exercises, or progressive muscle relaxation into your bedtime routine to help calm your mind and body before sleeping.

5. Consult Your Doctor: If you are struggling with sleep despite implementing these tips, consult your doctor as they may recommend medication or other treatments to help improve your sleep quality while dealing with leukaemia or a blood disorder.

In conclusion, getting enough quality sleep is crucial for managing the symptoms of leukaemia and blood disorders while optimising your lifestyle for overall health and wellbeing. By following these tips for improving sleep quality, you can enhance cognitive function, reduce fatigue, pain, anxiety, depression, and improve mood while dealing with these conditions. Remember always to consult with your healthcare provider regarding any medical concerns related to your condition or treatment plan before making any significant lifestyle changes or implementing new treatments or therapies into your routine!

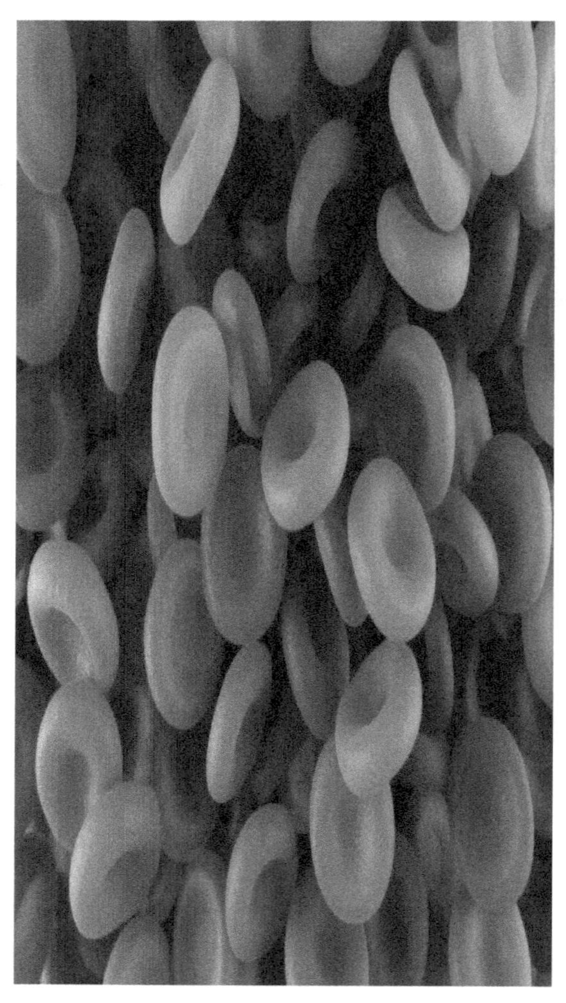

CHAPTER SIX

Coping with Emotional Challenges

Strategies for Emotional Well-being

Coping with a diagnosis of leukaemia or any other blood disease can be an emotionally challenging experience. The physical symptoms and treatments can take a toll on one's mental and emotional well-being, leading to feelings of anxiety, depression, and stress. However, there are strategies that individuals with leukaemia and blood diseases can adopt to manage their emotional challenges and promote emotional well-being.

1. Seek Support:

It's essential to have a support system in place during this challenging time. This could be family, friends, or a support group for people with leukaemia or blood diseases. Talking to others who understand what you're going through can provide comfort, encouragement, and practical advice.

2. Practice Mindfulness:

Mindfulness is a technique that involves focusing your attention on the present moment without judgement. It can help reduce stress, anxiety, and depression by promoting relaxation and self-awareness. Mindfulness meditation, deep breathing exercises, or yoga can be helpful in managing emotional challenges.

3. Stay Positive:

Maintaining a positive outlook can help individuals with leukaemia and blood diseases cope better with their emotional challenges. This involves focusing on the things that matter most, such as spending time with loved ones, pursuing hobbies or interests, and finding meaning and purpose in life despite the illness.

4. Manage Stress:

Stress is a common trigger for emotional challenges in individuals with leukaemia and blood diseases. Learning stress management techniques such as relaxation techniques, exercise, or therapy can help manage stress levels and promote emotional well-being.

5. Communicate Effectively:

Communication is essential in managing emotional challenges during treatment for leukaemia or blood diseases. Patients should communicate openly and honestly with their healthcare providers about their concerns, fears, and expectations regarding treatment options and outcomes. This can help them make informed decisions about their care and manage their emotions better.

6. Take Care of Yourself:

Self-care is crucial in managing emotional challenges during treatment for leukaemia or blood diseases. This involves taking care of one's physical health by eating healthy foods, getting enough sleep, and exercising regularly. Self-care also involves engaging in activities that bring joy and pleasure, such as reading a book, watching a movie, or listening to music.

7. Seek Professional Help:

If emotional challenges become overwhelming or interfere with daily functioning, seeking professional help from a mental health professional such as a psychologist or therapist can be beneficial. They can provide additional support, coping strategies, and resources to manage emotional challenges during treatment for leukaemia or blood diseases.

In conclusion, coping with emotional challenges during treatment for leukaemia or blood diseases requires a multifaceted approach that includes seeking support, practising mindfulness, staying positive, managing stress, communicating effectively, taking care of oneself and getting professional assistance as necessary. By implementing these strategies, individuals with leukaemia and blood diseases can promote emotional well-being during this challenging time.

Building a Support System

Coping with emotional challenges is an essential part of managing leukaemia and blood diseases. The diagnosis and treatment process can be overwhelming, causing feelings of fear, anxiety, and depression. Building a support system can provide the necessary emotional and practical support to help individuals navigate through these challenges. Here are some ways to build a support system in coping with emotional challenges for leukaemia and blood diseases:

- Connect with healthcare professionals: Healthcare professionals such as oncologists, nurses, and social workers are trained to provide emotional support to patients. They can offer guidance on coping strategies, connect patients with support groups, and provide referrals to mental health professionals if needed.

- Join a support group: Support groups offer a safe and supportive environment for patients to share their experiences, fears, and concerns with others who understand what they are going through. These groups can provide practical advice, emotional support, and a sense of community.

- Lean on family and friends: Family and friends can offer practical and emotional support during treatment. They can help with transportation to appointments, prepare meals, or simply provide a listening ear. It's essential to communicate openly with loved ones about how they can best support the patient during this time.

- Utilise online resources: There are many online resources available for patients with leukaemia and blood diseases. Websites such as Leukaemia & Lymphoma NZ offer information on coping strategies, treatment options, and resources for emotional support. Online support groups can also be helpful for those who cannot attend in-person meetings due to distance or mobility issues.

- Practice self-care: Self-care is essential for managing emotional challenges during treatment. Patients should prioritise activities that bring them joy and relaxation, such as meditation, yoga, or reading a book. They should also communicate openly with their healthcare team about any concerns they have regarding their emotional wellbeing.

In conclusion, building a support system is crucial for managing emotional challenges during treatment for leukaemia and blood diseases. Patients should connect with healthcare professionals, join a support group, lean on family and friends, utilise online resources, and practice self-care to ensure they have the necessary emotional and practical support throughout their journey. By building a strong support system, patients can better cope with the emotional challenges that come with these diseases.

CONCLUSION

Prevention, Hope, and Conclusion

Healthy Habits for Prevention

Prevention is key when it comes to managing health conditions, and this is especially true for leukaemia and other blood diseases. While there is no guaranteed way to prevent these diseases, adopting healthy habits can significantly reduce the risk of developing them. In this article, we will discuss some healthy habits that can help prevent leukaemia and blood diseases.

Prevention:

1. Maintain a healthy weight: Being overweight or obese increases the risk of developing leukaemia and other blood diseases. This is because excess weight can lead to chronic inflammation, which has been linked to the development of these conditions. Maintaining a healthy weight through a balanced diet and regular exercise can help reduce inflammation and lower the risk of developing these diseases.

2. Quit smoking: Smoking is a major risk factor for leukaemia and other blood diseases. The chemicals in tobacco smoke can damage the bone marrow, which is where blood cells are produced.

This damage can lead to the development of leukaemia and other blood disorders. Quitting smoking can reduce the risk of developing these diseases greatly.

3. Limit alcohol consumption: Excessive alcohol consumption has been linked to an increased risk of developing leukaemia and other blood diseases. This is because alcohol can damage the bone marrow and disrupt the production of blood cells. Limiting alcohol consumption to reasonable levels (one drink per day for women and two drinks per day for men) can help minimise the chance of developing these diseases.

4. Protect yourself from infections: Certain viruses, such as the human immunodeficiency virus (HIV) and hepatitis B and C viruses, have been linked to an increased risk of developing leukaemia and other blood diseases. Protecting yourself from these infections by practising safe sex, getting vaccinated against hepatitis B, and avoiding exposure to contaminated blood or bodily fluids can help reduce the risk of developing these diseases.

5. Eat a healthy diet: Eating a diet rich in fruits, vegetables, whole grains, and lean protein can help reduce inflammation and lower the risk of developing leukaemia and other blood diseases. Foods that are high in antioxidants, such as berries, leafy greens, and nuts, can also help protect

against these conditions by neutralising free radicals that can damage cells in the bone marrow.

Hope:

While there is no cure for leukaemia or other blood diseases, there are treatments available that can help manage the condition and improve quality of life. Advances in medical research have led to new therapies that are more effective at treating these diseases with fewer side effects. Additionally, support groups and counselling services can provide emotional support and resources for patients and their families during this difficult time.

Conclusion:

Preventing leukaemia and other blood diseases through healthy habits is important, but it's also important to remember that these conditions are not always preventable. If you or a loved one has been diagnosed with a blood disease, it's important to work with a healthcare provider to develop a treatment plan that meets your individual needs. By staying informed about new treatments and resources available, you can take an active role in managing your condition and improving your quality of life. Remember that hope is always possible, even in the face of adversity.

Inspiring Success Stories

Leukaemia and blood diseases are some of the most challenging health issues that people face today. The diagnosis of these diseases can be devastating, leaving patients and their families feeling overwhelmed and uncertain about the future, and the treatment process can be long and arduous. However, there are inspiring success stories of individuals who have overcome these diseases through prevention, hope, and perseverance. In this article, we will explore some of these stories, the progress being made in the fight against leukaemia and blood diseases, and the lessons we can learn from them.

Prevention: The Importance of Early Detection

Prevention is always better than cure, and this is especially true when it comes to leukaemia and blood diseases. Early detection is crucial in preventing the progression of these diseases and improving the chances of successful treatment. One such success story is that of Chris Herren, a former professional basketball player who battled drug addiction and alcoholism for over a decade. In 2008, Chris was diagnosed with acute myeloid leukaemia (AML), a type of blood cancer. However, because the disease was caught early, Chris was able to undergo intensive chemotherapy and achieve remission within a few months. Today,

Chris is cancer-free and has dedicated his life to helping others overcome addiction and prevent health issues like leukaemia through early detection.

Researchers are making significant strides in preventing leukaemia and blood diseases. One such example is the discovery of a gene mutation that increases the risk of acute myeloid leukaemia (AML). This discovery has led to the development of a blood test that can detect the mutation in individuals who may be at risk of developing AML. By identifying these individuals early, doctors can monitor them closely and intervene before the disease progresses.

Another example of prevention is the use of stem cell transplants to treat certain blood diseases. Stem cell transplants involve replacing damaged or diseased stem cells with healthy ones, effectively curing the disease. Researchers are now exploring ways to use stem cell transplants to prevent blood diseases from developing in the first place. By replacing stem cells in individuals who are at high risk of developing a blood disease, doctors can potentially prevent the disease from ever occurring.

Hope: The Power of Positivity

There have been many hopeful developments in the treatment of leukaemia and blood diseases in recent years. One such development is the use of immunotherapy to treat these diseases.

Immunotherapy involves using a patient's own immune system to fight cancer cells. By harnessing the power of the immune system, doctors can target cancer cells more effectively than traditional chemotherapy or radiation therapy.

Hope is a powerful force that can help individuals overcome even the most challenging health issues. It gives them the strength to keep fighting, even when the odds seem stacked against them.

One such success story is that of Beth Caldwell, a mother of three who was diagnosed with chronic myeloid leukaemia (CML) in 2007. Beth's diagnosis came at a difficult time in her life, as she was also dealing with financial hardship and personal struggles. However, Beth refused to give up hope and instead chose to focus on her faith and her family. She underwent treatment for CML and has been in remission ever since. Today, Beth is an advocate for CML patients and helps others find hope in their own journeys with leukaemia and blood diseases.

Another promising development is the use of targeted therapies to treat leukaemia and blood diseases. Targeted therapies are designed to specifically target cancer cells, sparing healthy cells from harm. This approach has led to more effective treatments with fewer side effects than traditional chemotherapy or radiation therapy.

Perseverance is essential in overcoming leukaemia and blood diseases, as these diseases can be incredibly challenging to treat. It takes a tremendous amount of courage and determination to keep fighting, even when the road ahead seems long and difficult. One such success story is that of Sarah Cannon, a cancer survivor who was diagnosed with acute lymphoblastic leukaemia (ALL) in 2014 at the age of 34. Sarah's diagnosis came at a time when she was already dealing with personal challenges, including a recent divorce and financial hardship. However, Sarah refused to give up hope or let her circumstances define her. She underwent aggressive chemotherapy treatment for ALL and has been in remission ever since. Today, Sarah is an advocate for cancer patients and helps others find hope in their own journeys with leukaemia and blood diseases through her work as a patient navigator in Nashville, Tennessee, at the Sarah Cannon Cancer Institute.

Conclusion

While there is still much work to be done in the fight against leukaemia and blood diseases, there have been many inspiring success stories in prevention, hope, and conclusion. From preventing diseases through early detection and stem cell transplants to treating them with immunotherapy and targeted therapies, researchers are making significant strides in improving outcomes for patients with these diseases. As research continues, we can hope for even more breakthroughs that will lead to better prevention, treatment, and ultimately, a cure for leukaemia and blood diseases.

The success stories of Chris Herren, Beth Caldwell, and Sarah Cannon teach us several valuable lessons about prevention, hope, and perseverance when it comes to leukaemia and blood diseases. Firstly, early detection is crucial in preventing the progression of these diseases and improving the chances of successful treatment. Secondly, hope is a powerful force that can help individuals overcome even the most challenging health issues. Thirdly, perseverance is essential in overcoming leukaemia and blood diseases, as these diseases can be incredibly challenging to treat. By learning from these success stories and applying their lessons to our own lives, we can all take steps towards preventing leukaemia and blood diseases, finding hope in our own journeys with these diseases, and persevering through the challenges they present us with.

Encouragement and Hope

Prevention:

Leukaemia and other blood diseases are often caused by genetic factors, environmental exposures, or lifestyle choices. While there is no guaranteed way to prevent these diseases, there are steps that individuals can take to reduce their risk.

Firstly, avoiding exposure to known carcinogens such as tobacco smoke, radiation, and certain chemicals can help prevent the development of blood diseases. Secondly, maintaining a healthy weight and engaging in regular exercise can help reduce the risk of obesity, which has been linked to an increased risk of leukaemia. Thirdly, getting vaccinated against hepatitis B and C viruses, which can lead to liver damage and increase the risk of developing blood diseases, is recommended. Fourthly, practicing safe sex and getting tested for sexually transmitted infections (STIs) can help prevent the transmission of HIV, which can weaken the immune system and increase the risk of developing blood diseases.

Hope:

While there is currently no cure for leukaemia and other blood diseases, there are promising developments in research that offer hope for the future. Advances in gene therapy, immunotherapy, and targeted therapies have shown promising results in clinical trials, leading to new treatments that are more effective and less toxic than traditional chemotherapy.

For example, CAR T-cell therapy involves genetically modifying a patient's own immune cells to target and destroy cancer cells. This therapy has shown remarkable success in treating certain types of leukaemia and lymphoma, with some patients experiencing complete remission. Similarly, CRISPR-Cas9 gene editing technology has the potential to correct genetic mutations that cause blood diseases at their source, offering a more permanent solution than traditional treatments.

In conclusion, while leukaemia and other blood diseases are still a major health concern, there is reason for hope. By taking steps to prevent these diseases through lifestyle choices and avoiding known carcinogens, individuals can reduce their risk. Additionally, ongoing research into new treatments such as CAR T-cell therapy and CRISPR-Cas9 gene editing offers promising developments for the future. While there is still much work to be done in this field, the progress made so far provides hope for a brighter future for those affected by these devastating diseases.

9 798887 268273